This is My Story

❁ STEPHEN L. FRITZ ❁

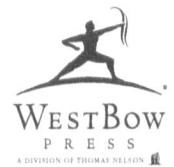

WESTBOW
PRESS
A DIVISION OF THOMAS NELSON

WestBow Press books may be ordered through booksellers or by contacting:

WestBow Press
A Division of Thomas Nelson
1663 Liberty Drive
Bloomington, IN 47403
www.westbowpress.com
1-(866) 928-1240

Because of the dynamic nature of the Internet, any web addresses or links contained in this book may have changed since publication and may no longer be valid. The views expressed in this work are solely those of the author and do not necessarily reflect the views of the publisher, and the publisher hereby disclaims any responsibility for them.

Any people depicted in stock imagery provided by Thinkstock are models, and such images are being used for illustrative purposes only.

Certain stock imagery © Thinkstock.

ISBN: 978-1-4497-2506-8 (sc)
ISBN: 978-1-4497-2505-1 (e)

Library of Congress Control Number: 2011914747

Printed in the United States of America

WestBow Press rev. date: 9/15/2011

To My Wife

As I write this I recall the many times that Ruth expressed to me her longing to minister to women who were going through difficult times.

God works in so many ways. While Ruth was going through her cancer treatment she was doing the very thing that she so wanted to do—inspiring and lifting up all those around her.

Many pastors from different congregations visited and prayed with Ruth but they never left without Ruth praying for them. In fact she took great joy in taking the time to pray for her friends, family, doctors, nurses and every person who came to see her. She inspired the very people who were coming to help her.

Through *This Is My Story* Ruth tells us that the strength which the Lord Jesus provides is given freely. And with this strength we as Christians can overcome the difficulties that life lays at our feet.

Ruth's story is dedicated not only to struggling women but also to all who will come to know the Power and Glory of our Lord and Savior Jesus Christ.

Stephen L. Fritz

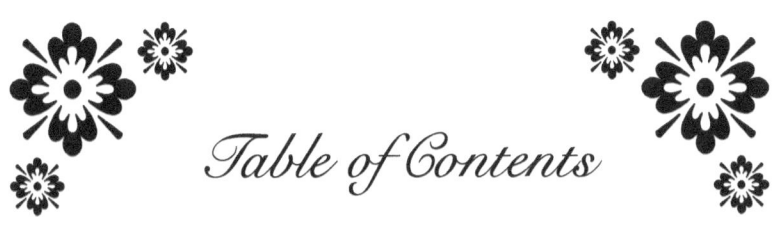

Table of Contents

Preface

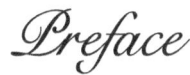

Most people have heard the saying, God works in mysterious ways. And by most accounts this story is a prime example. My name is Stephen. Ruth was my wife for nearly fourteen years and we have an eleven year old daughter Estefany. Ruth's story for me begins about two years before her passing. Ruth would tell me of how she felt God had put on her heart to write a book for the support of women in their search for spiritual growth. Ruth wanted to focus on women who were struggling and not just those who were going through cancer but anyone who was struggling with life's hardships.

Several years ago Ruth shared her thoughts and desires for this project. Although I listened, I wondered how Ruth could write a book when she was barely able to sit in a chair for more than 20 minutes without being in severe pain. So I listened with an open heart and mind while still thinking how this could ever happen. As the days passed by slowly, Ruth's condition became worse. On July 18th Ruth went to meet her Lord and Savior, Jesus Christ. Now you might think this is the closing of a chapter of pain and suffering and final victory going to meet God in heaven but Ruth and God hadn't completed their work. *This Is My Story* had not been written.

Almost every morning Ruth would awaken with pain and discomfort between 2 and 3 in the morning. So I was used to getting up and checking on her, doing what needed to be done, then trying to go back to bed. Then a week or two after Ruth's passing between 2 and 3 AM I awoke with an urgent need to write. But I didn't want to write and it seemed that I had an argument with Ruth and God the rest of the night. I told them that there was no way I could write Ruth's book—not me! Find a real author who has already written books. I've been a musician for forty year and have written hundreds of sounds, different genres, and even some Christian songs, but a book—never!

As you can see, I didn't win that argument. So began my first venture into writing a book. As with composing a song, at times I had to step back from the keyboard and take time to reflect. The book was inspired by the Holy Spirit, not by my abilities or anything I could bring to words. Ruth's story was one of faith, strength and courage which she gave to all of us around her. She wanted others to know where her strength and hope came from.

God uses difficult situations to draw us closer to Him. Many times we don't understand why this is happening. God has a plan and one day we will know the reasons why. Seek to find your strength in God's promise and His internal gift through Jesus Christ, God's only Son, who died that you may have eternal life. *This Is My Story.*

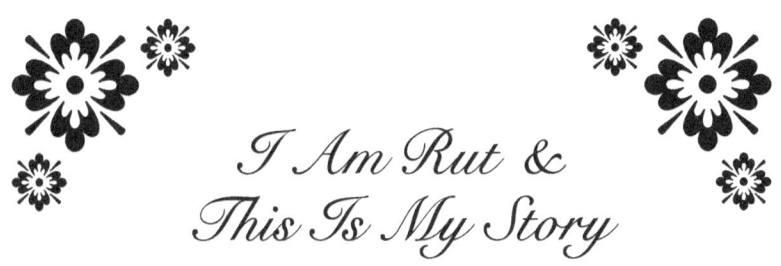

I Am Rut & This Is My Story

I am Rut and this is my story . . . On May 5th 1969 I was born Rut* Dored Rodriguez on the island of Puerto Rico. (After moving to Indiana I changed my name to Ruth.) My mother and father Dorcus and Eduardo Rodriguez raised me along with my sister Debra and brother Wardie. Mommy stayed at home and Daddy went off to work through the week. We all attended church on Sunday and through the week when there were activities. We were raised like so many other Christian children in the church today.

I remember singing at a very early age. Without any formal lessons I had been blessed with the ability to sing. When I got older I was called by the Holy Spirit to use His gift of singing.

I sang with a small group of my friends at church. Often we had the opportunity to sing and give our testimonies at other churches. This was a wonderful experience which I treasured all of my life.

I hope this small book will inspire you to seek God's plan for your life. I know that in my journey Jesus shielded me with His love and kindness. He comforted me in the beginning and walked with me till the end. I am now resting in His arms.

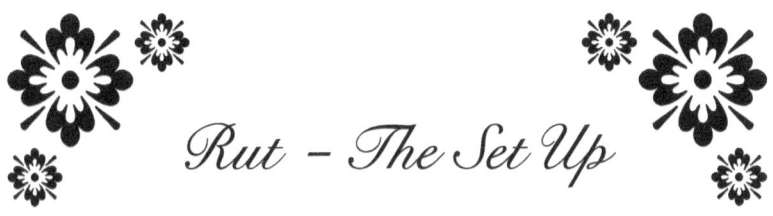

Rut – The Set Up

I believe we know as individuals when the Holy Spirit is talking to our hearts. Even when our lives aren't what they should be, God is there.

When you have given your heart to the Lord, you don't come back later and say, "I want it back." It's not that simple. You can't run and you can't hide from the Word and truth that God has given you and put on your heart and in your mind.

Isaiah 55:11 (NIV)

[11] My word that goes out from my mouth: It will not return to me empty, but will accomplish what I desire and achieve the purpose for which I sent it.

Once you have started to plow the field of righteousness and have begun your journey with the Lord, it has been written that it would be better for a man never to start plowing the field than to stop and return to his old ways.

God has received so many of us back into His loving arms after we have turned away from Him for a season. Praise God for His mercy and goodness.

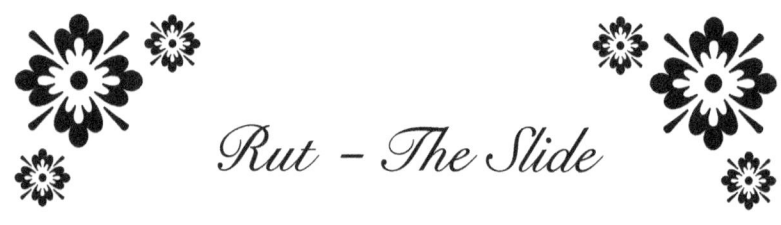

Rut – The Slide

Let me take a little time to explain what started my backward slide away from God. It happens to so many of us. We follow our heart's desires and close our eyes and ears to the voice of the Holy Spirit.

I found myself looking for freedom. We all search to control our lives while trying to show ourselves and everyone else that we already have control of our lives.

My search for control started in my twenties. I was going to school to become a special education teacher for Down's syndrome children. I still was attending church and singing but it was becoming a little less all the time. This is the process that slowly moves us away from what we know is right.

I was teaching and I had my own car and apartment. By the world's standards I had it all. I even had a handsome boyfriend who was studying to be a lawyer.

What else could a girl need or want? But I was missing something. It seemed God was pulling me one way and I just kept pulling back the other way. Maybe I was missing a husband. Getting married to this wonderful man was what I needed. I could live happily ever after and this would surely complete my happiness.

So I did it; I got married. We enjoyed the big wedding with family and friends. It just seemed like I was in control now and everything was going my way.

Then one day I received a call from one of my best friends. She said, "Come to the mall now." She didn't say why but just said, "Don't waste any time." So I rushed to the mall to meet her. She grabbed my hand and headed for the food court where she pointed to a table below and said, "Isn't that your husband with that girl?" My heart was thrown into ten different directions all at once. I walked to the table and said it's over, threw down my ring, and walked away. My control had just been taken from my hands!

The words I spoke 'it's over' were really just the beginning of a divorce in the making. It was not pleasant as many of them are not. But when two people are not together for the right reasons and without the guidance of a greater purpose with a good foundation, all other ground is sinking sand.

What was I thinking? OK so I got out of that one—notice I said 'I'. Then I started down a new road of real confusion. It wasn't long till I found myself involved with another man. He ran a Glamour Shots Store in the mall. That should have been a clue. By now I was really running from the truth. I knew it so well but didn't want to embrace it. This relationship promised excitement and adventure and traveling to distant cities. Who in their right mind would pass that by? Not me. I wasn't the one who would be left behind on this adventure.

So before I could say 'flyaway' three times I found myself in Evansville. For those of you who don't know anything about Indiana, I'm here to tell you that it's not Puerto Rico. I was asked so many times why I was in Indiana when Puerto Rico was one of the most beautiful places on the planet. I had to agree. Puerto Rico is very beautiful but I was here for adventure and a longing for love.

Little did I know my choice of men just wasn't too keen. It seemed I had an extraordinary ability to choose these not so faithful men. Once again I found myself hurt, used, and left with this emptiness. But God was working on my come back.

God was working on what I could not achieve on my own. He was starting to call me home into His fellowship. At the same time God was working in a man's life—the man I would eventually marry. This man was going through the same things I had been going through. He had also had relationship problems. And like me, so many of his choices were without prayer. But finally he started praying for that perfect match. That was me—he just didn't know it yet.

I returned to Puerto Rico but not before a friend talked to me about a man named Steve whom I had already met on several occasions.

Steve seemed happy and carefree. I can't say at that time I knew there was or could be a connection; however, he did seem nice. But so much was still going on and getting out is so much harder than jumping in. Life was getting more complex, especially with me running things. I was running out of ideas. So I got back on a plane to Puerto Rico.

Maybe I could find my direction once again. I was there two weeks with thoughts of not returning to Indiana. But there was something that my friend in Indiana said about Steve. He really liked me a lot and would love to spend time with me. I felt drawn to Evansville. That seemed so much different than 'you're beautiful and I just have to have you.' I didn't want to be had.

My mind was made up and I must say with some prayer, although I wasn't sure how far that was going to go with all the space I had been putting between myself and the Lord.

When I arrived in Evansville, a friend and I went to one of the properties Steve owned and was managing. I asked my friend to go in and tell him that I came back and wanted to talk. A few minutes passed. Then he came out and greeted me with open arms. At that moment I knew he was the one. There was something special in his face and his smile. I felt we had been together for a very long time. But we had only started our journey and what a journey it became!

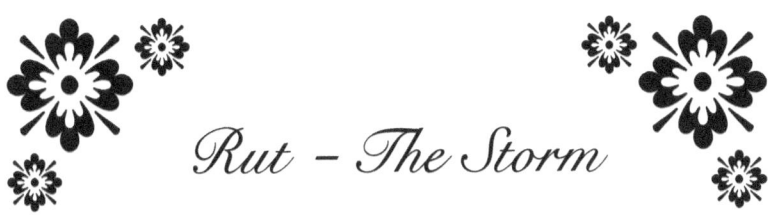

Rut – The Storm

As early as about 1997 I felt physically something just wasn't right. I never could identify the problem but I began going to the doctor more and having tests run. Everything came back OK. Then after my pregnancy I started having more problems. Again I visited the doctor and they ran tests and again found nothing.

There were times pain would come over me; my heart would race and Steve would take me to the hospital. After two or three visits to the emergency room I began driving myself when problems arose. No one could believe there was anything really wrong with me. We had no insurance and the bills mounted. I felt I was causing such a burden on our family.

There were times I would start feeling better and think it was going to be all right. My gynecologist and I decided I should have a partial hysterectomy. I had this surgery which went well, but it wasn't long until I had more problems.

Once again I went back to my gynecologist for a checkup. I asked Steve to go in with me and he did. My doctor performed the exam and said everything looked normal. I was stunned when she mentioned I might need to see someone for an emotional problem. Steve might have thought the same at the time but later told me he was so sorry for even thinking that to be true. He realized I was someone who knew my body and there was something wrong.

Shortly after that last check up Steve and I insisted the doctor go in and take a biopsy. When the biopsy came back it showed I had a very rare type of cervical cancer.

Unsure of my future I was scared but relieved to know my problem. Mostly I was scared for my family, my daughter, and my husband. I knew I had a path of chemo, radiation, and possible surgery. This was as bad as it could get—or so I thought.

My first appointment was with a specialist in Indianapolis, Indiana. Who would have thought the guru of this rare cancer would be in Indiana? God works in mysterious ways.

He told us that going through chemo and radiation reduced the cancer but surgery would still be needed. We were told that the cancer could have been detected earlier by a trained eye. The thought of this was so big I could hardly get my mind around it. Steve went on the internet and read and printed the whole process I would have to endure. He asked me if I needed to know anything about this surgery, as it meant removing a lot of internal organs and much more. I declined the information, knowing it wasn't going to make it easier.

I now had a little insight on how Jesus felt in the garden when He cried to the Father about the cup He needed to drink. That had to be more than any short felt problem I had. For three nights I cried in my closet and asked God to spare me for just a little longer. I made up my mind to wrap myself in a Shield of Faith and to worship Him in song until I couldn't get up from the bed.

After five years of living with this cancer, my life had been changed. My husband and many of my friends had also changed. My daughter was growing and becoming a beautiful girl and I prayed that she would always remember how much I loved her. She had been an inspiration to my life in more ways than she would ever know. I would never forget seeing her in church dancing like an angel to Jesus and worshipping Him in praise.

Once she told me that a person was so mean to her and she was so tired of that. I told her to tell Jesus about those things. He could work everything out. I prayed she would always follow this good lesson.

My husband helped me with my courage and God gave me what I needed. It wasn't always what I wanted but I learned not to compare with what someone else had but to be thankful for my blessings. I knew there was great need in the world and the community. We needed to stand strong and work as the time was near and there was so much to do.

God held me in His hands for many years. He blessed me with a loving husband, a wonderful daughter, supportive family, and so many wonderful riches I could only thank Him! It was said with my cancer I should never have become pregnant with a child and I did. It was said I should not live past thirty and I did. I went home at the age of forty one.

I WOULD LIKE TO LEAVE YOU
WITH SOME OF MY FAVORITE SCRIPTURES:

Hebrews 10:35-39 (NIV)

[35]So do not throw away your confidence; it will be richly rewarded.

[36]You need to persevere so that when you have done the will of God, you will receive what he has promised.

[37]For in just a very little while, "He who is coming will come and will not delay.

[38]But my righteous one will live by faith. And if he shrinks back, I will not be pleased with him."

[39]But we are not of those who shrink back and are destroyed, but of those who believe and are saved.

Luke 18:35-43 (NIV)

[35]As Jesus approached Jericho, a blind man was sitting by the roadside begging.

[36]When he heard the crowd going by, he asked what was happening.

[37]They told him, "Jesus of Nazareth is passing by."

[38]He called out, "Jesus, Son of David, have mercy on me!"

[39]Those who led the way rebuked him and told him to be quiet, but he shouted all the more, "Son of David, have mercy on me!"

[40]Jesus stopped and ordered the man to be brought to him. When he came near, Jesus asked him,

[41]"What do you want me to do for you?" "Lord, I want to see," he replied.

[42]Jesus said to him, "Receive your sight; your faith has healed you."

[43]Immediately he received his sight and followed Jesus, praising God. When all the people saw it, they also praised God.

James 5:16 (NIV)

[16]Therefore confess your sins to each other and pray for each other so that you may be healed. The prayer of a righteous man is powerful and effective.

Galatians 3:14 (NIV)

[14]He redeemed us in order that the blessing given to Abraham might come to the Gentiles through Christ Jesus, so that by faith we might receive the promise of the Spirit.

Galatians 5:16 (NIV)

[16]So I say, live by the Spirit, and you will not gratify the desires of the sinful nature.

Proverbs 18:5-9 (NIV)

[5] It is not good to be partial to the wicked or to deprive the innocent of justice.

[6] A fool's lips bring him strife, and his mouth invites a beating.

[7] A fool's mouth is his undoing, and his lips are a snare to his soul.

[8] The words of a gossip are like choice morsels; they go down to a man's inmost parts.

[9] One who is slack in his work is brother to one who destroys.

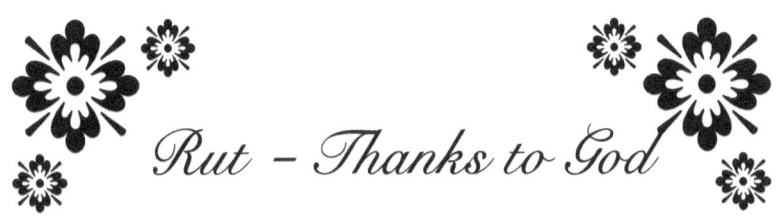

Rut – Thanks to God

Thanks to God for what He made
Thanks to God for me He saved
Thanks to God His son He gave
And died for me my soul to save
I'll praise Him through the night till day
I'll praise Him through my strife and pain
I know He holds me both day and night
I wait for Him as His child.

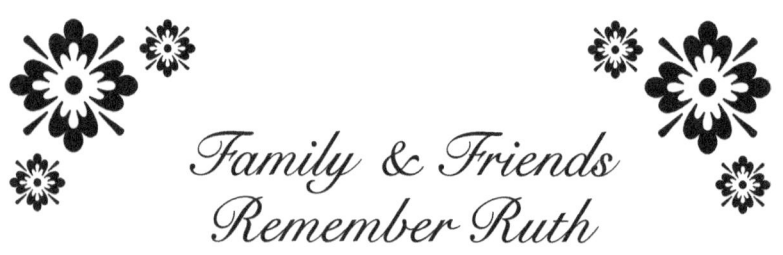

Family & Friends Remember Ruth

Steve remembers . . . I was married to Ruth for thirteen years. As with many couples we had our ups and downs. Ruth tells the story of our quest for companionship and love. A journey that ended at the foot of the cross . . . though many times we strayed from our redemptive love and the power of our Lord and Savior.

Ruth started her journey back to Jesus before she ever became aware of her disease. Jesus called her back into fellowship and at the same time He was working in my life. Ruth was the key element in not only my life but also in so many others. Her strength and faith held her up through the trials she was facing. And although Ruth cried many times with pain and fear throughout the five years that she battled this disease, the Lord always covered her with His love. Even as she was passing through the shadow of death, she gave God the glory and kept her eyes on Jesus who received her with open arms at the end of her earthly life.

Ruth will always be missed but never forgotten because of her love and concern for others. She wanted everyone to know the love of Jesus and to accept the Lord Jesus as their personal Savior.

I encourage you, your families and loved ones to find the peace which transcends all understanding. You can find the Lord in so many ways when you allow yourself to become open to the Holy Spirit. Let God be your shield and may you find comfort in the Lord when you are going through difficult trials and day to day challenges.

I hope you share this story with others, remembering that one day you will meet Ruth and all the others who went before at a reunion filled with joy and gladness. This is God's promise that we have through His son, Jesus Christ.

~ ~ ~ ~ ~ ~

Trudy remembers . . . Ruth inspired me with her courage. She had a way of making others feel so special. No matter what she was facing or what she had gone through that day, her focus was on the other person. She wanted to know what was happening in your world. And no matter what you told her, she made you feel like she was going to be getting well and would do her part to help you. She had a strong desire to help others and never gave up.

When the move to another house was necessary, Ruth picked colors and other items needed to decorate their home. That showed me that God uses us our whole journey in life and not just part of it.

One time while she was hospitalized one of her nurses was excited because her son was returning from Iraq. His first stop was going to be the hospital to see his mother. When he arrived, the nurse brought him in to see Ruth. After talking for awhile, Ruth had all of us move in close together and join hands to pray for him. She loved to pray and to have everyone close with hands joined together. And I always loved to hear Ruth pray. She prayed not just for this young soldier's safety but for the safety of all the other soldiers and to make their five senses alert to danger. She finished the prayer in her mother language which the soldier understood as he had studied Spanish.

God is so good. Ruth was blessed with many gifts which she generously shared with others. I felt special to be a part of her life. I saw how God worked in both Ruth and Stephen's lives and how he transformed them from a strong couple to a mother and father and then to a family involved in the community. Thank you both for letting me be a part of your lives.

~ ~ ~ ~ ~ ~

Heather remembers . . .
"As the heavens are higher than the earth, so are my
ways higher than your ways and my thoughts than your
thoughts." Isaiah 55:9

Thank you Ruth for your walk of faith. I continue to exercise
my faith. And when it is hard and challenging, I think of you
and am inspired to give it to God and speak in faith.

It is hard to convey in just a few words what Ruth meant to me
and what her impact here on earth continues to be on me and
on many others. Whether you were a long time friend or a brief
acquaintance, she was outspoken in her faith and shared with
all what Jesus had done in her life and could do in theirs.

One time I called her while in my last days of being pregnant
with my oldest son. My due date was fast approaching and I
feared having a "C" section. I was very scared and disappointed
that I might not be able to experience natural childbirth. When
I spoke with Ruth, she was very strong about speaking in faith
and not speaking the worry and fear that had captured my
thoughts at that time.

It is such practical advice, "Speak in faith." Ruth always spoke
in faith even through her diagnosis, treatment, and in her final
days here on earth.

I am sure when you are close to meeting your King the motivation to "just do it" certainly resonates in all actions, thoughts and motivations. With Ruth it came from a place of ease and certainty and not from a place of 'I am on a tight schedule here; my life may be coming to a close.' Her prayers came from a place of faith, Godly faith. Ruth lived her faith and spoke faith to those in her life.

This lesson of how to exercise faith is what she has branded on my life—to not speak the insecurities of my mind that arise in the situations I face daily. Instead I focus on Isaiah 55:9 and exercise the faith I have in God to carry me through, no matter how large or small the problem. I now give it to God because He holds me, and His plans for me are amazing. He holds the life of so many, including my family, my sister, my dad, my aunt, my mom and all those who have accepted Jesus as their Lord and Savior.

~ ~ ~ ~ ~ ~

Steve's mom remembers . . . If I were a great writer maybe, just maybe, the words would come to tell you about Ruth. She was an angel in disguise to our family.

I knew her first as my daughter-in-law. That was sudden and she didn't speak my language nor could I speak Spanish. But she spoke the language of love and kindness and made my son a happy man—and a better man. So I began to love her. Little did we know what the next years would bring . . .

First there was a very precious baby girl who was beautiful like her mother. What a gift! But then within the next three years Ruth began to develop health problems. She fought the fight with courage, faith in God and grace. The weaker her body became, the stronger her faith and the greater her love for God.

The last year was so amazing—in and out of hospitals, home for a week then the ambulance would take her away again. Her beautiful hair was gone and her body was so thin and fragile. I was afraid she would break. But . . . her faith, her love of her God—well that just got stronger and stronger.
So did she change me? Oh yes! Did I love her and miss her? Positively! Heaven is closer to me because Ruth is there. *I love you.*

⸝ ⸝ ⸝ ⸝ ⸝ ⸝

Jamie remembers . . . Steve, Ruth's husband, is my brother, one of three. When I first met Ruth in 1997, my first impression of her was that she was a beautiful, outgoing, and strong woman. She was so charismatic. My biggest challenge was getting her to slow her speech so I could understand her English. Ruth was easy for me to love right away because she loved family. And our family became her family since hers was in Puerto Rico. I had a new sister.

My Christian journey was similar to Ruth's so we had a lot in common. I was brought up in the Baptist Church. Our parents were teachers in the church and we went to church every time the doors were open. I learned about Jesus when I was very young and was baptized when I was 7 years old. I sang in the youth choir and went on summer choir trips to churches in the south and all around the Midwest. I loved my church friends and singing. However, unlike Ruth, I was the kid in Sunday school that asked, "Why and how do you know?" after every bible story. I wasn't easy to teach because of my doubting Thomas attitude, yet I knew the feeling that "Jesus came into my heart" was real and I prayed. Despite being saved, I was not sure about freewill, why there was a hell and why we were supposed to fear God. I was definitely conflicted.

As I became a young adult I, like Ruth, thought I could program my life to "my standard," which was part God and part world. I partied too much but I didn't want to turn "that part" of my life over to God. Bottom line, I didn't want God telling me who to date or what to do on that date. I wanted control.

As my business life grew, my personal life spun out of control. I was so unhappy. One minute God was lifting me up and the next I was doing my own thing. I had a strong desire to become successful on my own. I knew that if I could become successful, make money and live in the largest and most desirable cities I could have earthly happiness. My goal was the kind of success and happiness that is shown in TV commercials, movies and in magazines and provides earthly security. What could beat that?

As the years went by, my career and income topped even my wildest dreams. Then a drastic thing happened. While working, I became ill. In 1996 I developed fibromyalgia and soon after chronic fatigue syndrome. I continued to work but later was diagnosed with multiple allergies, asthma and arthritis. Because I was in poor health, the company I was working for fired me, years before I was financially prepared to retire and with no hope of replacing my job with another in the same field. I was in crisis. How was I going to pay the bills and raise my daughter? I knew that God had a plan for us if I could just give it over to Him. After two years of no income, huge insurance and drug bills, and many doctors, I was medically approved for Social Security Disability income. What an answer to prayer! How God took care of us!

Most of these years of obtaining my early desires I continued to go to church and live one foot in and one foot out of the true biblical Word from God. But my parents continued to pray for me. My father gave me *The Living Bible* marked with 2 Timothy 3:15 which says, "You know how, when you were a small child, you were taught the Holy Scriptures; and it is these that make you wise to accept God's salvation by trusting in Christ Jesus."

When Ruth became so sick she had to enter the hospital for what became the last 9 months of her life, with God's help I committed to be with her or assist her in any way I could. We spent countless hours watching movies, talking and sometimes napping. If she saw a commercial on TV for chicken nuggets or a slushy and she wanted it, I went and got it. Ruth never wavered from knowing how much God loved her and could heal her. She had a positive attitude even through violent days and nights of illness. All along I thought that *I* was helping *her*. Little did I know she would help me more than anyone ever had before.

What did I learn from Ruth? The full grasp of LOVE including her love for her child, husband, family and friends. But most importantly, I felt and saw the LOVE of GOD. When I was in the room with Ruth, whether feeding her, helping to change her bed or just watching TV, the overwhelming grace and love around her was awe inspiring. You could not miss it. Ruth would greet nurses, doctors and visitors with "How are you today?" Ruth prayed beautiful prayers for each of her visitors and hospital personnel and they in turn left feeling uplifted. God's love spoke so loudly through Ruth that even I (a doubting Thomas) couldn't miss it.

God works in mysterious ways! He knows how to reach people that have a desire to know Him and He does not let go of them. He wants every one of us to join Him for eternity in heaven, in love. This is what I learned from Ruth—from our first meeting until her death.

I know God has a plan for me today. I am in a women's bible group that feeds me with God's Word and I am growing spiritually by studying the bible. I miss Ruth terribly and I wish I could once again talk with her about her faith and her gift of ministering to people for Jesus. Ruth was a light to His world. She is my Christian example that God can use us at any time for His purpose.

Now I can say in truth that "I'm all in" for God! I fully trust Him and His redeeming love—a doubting Thomas no more!

~ ~ ~ ~ ~ ~

Ruth's father remembers . . . While living in Puerto Rico, Ruth had a car and a good job as a special education teacher. So her decision to move to Indiana came as a surprise to us especially since she did not speak good English. Although as parents we were not comfortable with her decision, we knew that our Lord Jesus Christ would take care of her.

She met Steve her future husband and they were later married. Her mother traveled to the US about once a year to visit and

Ruth came back to Puerto Rico occasionally to visit. All went well until 2006 when Ruth was diagnosed with cancer. Subsequently her mother and I traveled as much as we could to Indiana to spend time with our daughter and her family. Prayers and hymns were plentiful and seemed to soothe her pain.

Then on September 18, 2009 we learned that Ruth was not doing well. Her mother and I immediately left for Indiana. Our church held us up in prayer and put us in God's hands. Ruth was so thin and all the medication she was taking caused her to lose her appetite. We worked with her encouraging her to eat and she improved somewhat. Ruth spoke health for her body and declared a spirit of life to her body. She claimed health.

I accompanied the rest of the family to Ruth's appointment with the doctor who seemed somewhat surprised to see so many people. Afterwards with the help of an interpreter, I was able to speak to the doctor alone and was told that my daughter had stage four cancer which was terminal. He estimated that she only had six months to a year left to live. I was extremely shaken by that information but told him that God had the last word.

Ruth began her second round of chemotherapy which was much worse than the first—pain, vomiting, diarrhea, and hair falling out. She spent six days in the hospital.

I remembered Romans 8:28 (NIV)—"And we know that in all things God works for the good of those who love him, who have been called according to his purpose."

Ruth continued to remain positive and claim health for her body. And I thought, "Can this be SUPER faith or positive thinking—where is the reality? We are seeing a condition and its effects. But God is Sovereign and has the last word. I cited the Word where Paul begs God to remove the sting and God says, 'I give you my grace.'"

Philippians 4:6 (NIV) "Do not be anxious about anything, but in every situation, by prayer and petition, with thanksgiving, present your requests to God."

The Lord began to work with me. I started to get up at 3 AM to pray and intercede for Ruth.

On one of my visits to the hospital I was able to witness to a young man with cancer who had left his church and was having inappropriate relationships with women. He allowed me to pray for him and talk with him about Christ and His love. I saw him on two different days. The second time I saw him he told me that he had reconciled with the Lord and planned to return to church. Even during this most difficult time the Lord had allowed me to minister to this young man.

In one of the hospital waiting rooms there was a piano. And a gentleman about my age came in, sat down and began playing, "How Great Thou Art." I felt the presence of the Lord giving me strength and filling me with His joy and His peace . . . PRAISE THE LORD!

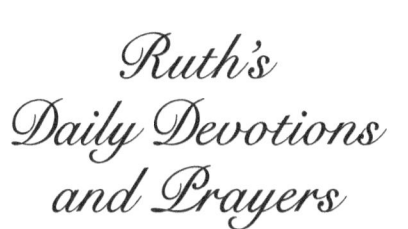

Ruth's Daily Devotions and Prayers

I have to forget myself and understand that God has forgiven me, and he loves me for who I am.

1 John 3:15-16 (NIV)

[15] Anyone who hates a brother or sister is a murderer, and you know that no murderer has eternal life residing in him.

[16] This is how we know what love is: Jesus Christ laid down his life for us. And we ought to lay down our lives for our brothers and sisters.

Let His love flow and show His love to others by your actions. Shut down criticism towards others and focus on Jesus and His love.

1 John 4:12 (NIV)

[12] No one has ever seen God; but if we love one another, God lives in us and His love is made complete in us.

When we can see God and His love, it can complement and work on the love we share with others.

We so many times are thinking of what's to be, and forget about others.

We say, you hurt me, you forgot me, and you disrespected me. We need to stop and understand God's perfect love. It can fulfill us.

He went to the cross and died for me. I just want to love like Jesus loves me.

Oh Lord I love you, and I need you. You are there all the time and always when I need you. Your love is patient and kind and I feel the love You provide.

Love doesn't keep a record, love is kind, and love doesn't expect everyone to adapt their life around what we want.

We serve God for His GLORY not ours.
Release my flesh so I can receive You—a perfect spirit.

Colossians 3:12-14 (NIV)

[12] Therefore, as God's chosen people, holy and dearly loved, clothe yourselves with compassion, kindness, humility, gentleness and patience.

¹³ Bear with each other and forgive one another if any of you has a grievance against someone. Forgive as the Lord forgave you.

¹⁴ And over all these virtues put on love, which binds them all together in perfect unity.

Love is more than a feeling, it's a responsibility. It's a behavior that will glorify His name.

Help me with my temper and the accepting of people that have another way. Help me to resist bad decisions, and help me to love others.

Lord help me, I don't want to feel upset when I don't get my way. Guard me from selfishness.

James 1:19-20 (NIV)
Listening and Doing

¹⁹ My dear brothers and sisters, take note of this: Everyone should be quick to listen, slow to speak and slow to become angry,

²⁰ because human anger does not produce the righteousness that God desires.

Listen and be still.

Proverbs 29:11 (NIV)

[11] Fools give full vent to their rage, but the wise bring calm in the end.

Yours is the GLORY and the HONOR. I lift up my hands and worship, and glorify Your name. You are great and do marvelous things, and there is no other like You.

God is Divine and He knows my needs. He shows me day by day how I can change and be ready for life each day.

I will ask my husband to pray for me today.

I pray to summit to my husband in God's love and grace.

He is our helper and desires only good things for us.

Bring me the passion of your Holy Spirit, and to recognize your living sacrifice.

Romans 12:1-2 (NIV)

A Living Sacrifice

[1] Therefore, I urge you, brothers and sisters, in view of God's mercy, to offer your bodies as a living sacrifice, holy and pleasing to God—this is your true and proper worship.

[2] Do not conform to the pattern of this world, but be transformed by the renewing of your mind. Then you will be able to test and approve what God's will is—his good, pleasing and perfect will.

He is a Holy God. He is the living water and we needed His sacrifice. He is looking for vessels, people that will surrender their lives to Him.

I love You so much, oh Lord. I am your vessel. Use me even though my body is failing.

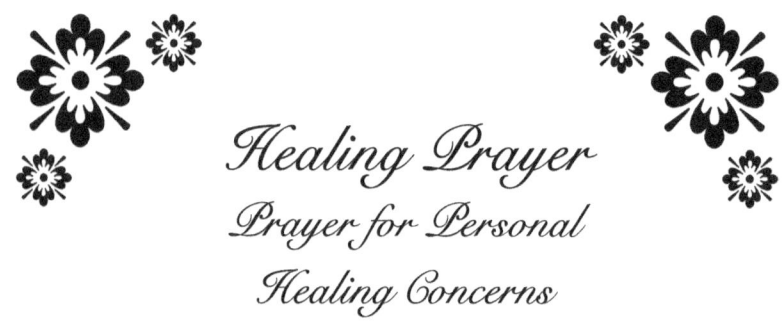

Healing Prayer
Prayer for Personal Healing Concerns

Ruth felt that people needed tools to guide them when praying for personal healing concerns. She wanted not only this book but especially this chapter to be a guide. In fact during the last year of her life she asked Steve to use this prayer and these scriptures each morning as he prayed.

Father God, in the Name of Jesus Christ, my Lord and Savior, I thank You that according to Your Word and my prayers, I walk in divine health <u>now</u>. I confess that all of Your promises concerning health and healing are Yes and in Christ, Amen, to the glory of God through me. Your Word declares that believers overcome the trials and the horrors of life through accepting the redeeming blood of Jesus as a completed work for them and the Word of their testimony or confession. Therefore, I confess the following concerning me and my health and what You in Your Word have declared as <u>forever settled</u>:

I believe, so I therefore declare and decree:

²⁴ "He himself bore our sins" in his body on the cross, so that we might die to sins and live for righteousness; "by his wounds you have been healed."
(I Peter 2:24 NIV)

¹⁷ This was to fulfill what was spoken through the prophet Isaiah:
"He took up our infirmities and bore our diseases."
(Matthew 8:17 NIV)

²⁰ My son, pay attention to what I say; turn your ear to my words.
²¹ Do not let them out of your sight, keep them within your heart;
²² for they are life to those who find them and health to one's whole body.
²³ Above all else, guard your heart, for everything you do flows from it.
(Proverbs 4:20-23 NIV)

I believe, so I therefore declare and decree:

⁴⁵ Not one of all the LORD's good promises to Israel failed; every one was fulfilled.
(Joshua 21:45 NIV)

¹¹ And if the Spirit of him who raised Jesus from the dead is living in you, he who raised Christ from the dead will also give life to your mortal bodies because of his Spirit who lives in you.
(Romans 8:11 NIV)

¹³ for it is God who works in you to will and to act in order to fulfill his good purpose.
(Philippians 2:13 NIV)

I believe, so I therefore declare and decree:

¹ Praise the LORD, my soul; all my inmost being, praise his holy name.
² Praise the LORD, my soul, and forget not all his benefits—
³ who forgives all your sins and heals all your diseases,
⁴ who redeems your life from the pit and crowns you with love and compassion,
⁵ who satisfies your desires with good things so that your youth is renewed like the eagle's.
(Psalms 103:1-5 NIV)

²⁰ He sent out his word and healed them; he rescued them from the grave.
(Psalms 107:20 NIV)

¹⁷ But I will restore you to health and heal your wounds,'
declares the LORD, 'because you are called an outcast, Zion
for whom no one cares.'
(Jeremiah 30:17 NIV)

I believe, so I therefore declare and decree:

¹⁹ This day I call the heavens and the earth as witnesses against
you that I have set before you life and death, blessings and
curses. Now choose life, so that you and your children may
live
(Deuteronomy 30:19 NIV)

⁹ Whatever they plot against the LORD he will bring to an
end; trouble will not come a second time.
(Nahum1:9 NIV)

¹³ Christ redeemed us from the curse of the law by becoming
a curse for us, for it is written: "Cursed is everyone who is
hung on a pole."
(Galatians 3:13 NIV)

I believe, so I therefore declare and decree:

¹⁷ Every good and perfect gift is from above, coming down
from the Father of the heavenly lights, who does not change
like shifting shadows.
(James 1:17 NIV)

Sickness in my body or in my mind is not from God. I receive the perfect gift of Life and Health in Christ Jesus. It is Your perfect will so I thank You for it. Glory to God!

I take full authority over you, Satan and I bind you and <u>all</u> your demons, in the Name of the Lord Jesus Christ! I <u>command</u> you to turn loose of my body <u>NOW</u>, and take your disease with you! You are under <u>my</u> feet and the blood of Jesus is <u>against</u> you!

I thank you Lord God, that Satan and his demons are bound and that they have NO authority over me or my body or my health. I thank You for providing for my every need and that includes wellness from the top of my head to the soles of my feet.

I thank You Father that I wear the whole armor of God, and that the Word and the shield of Faith protect me. To You, Father God, be all the Glory, Honor and Praise in Jesus' Mighty Name. Amen.

〃 〃 〃 〃 〃 〃

Pray this out <u>loud</u> every day, and allow the Word being confessed unto God to develop faith in you.

Romans 10:17 (NKJV)

[17] So then faith *comes* by hearing, and hearing by the word of God.

Read it aloud to your body just as if you were taking a medical prescription: <u>minimum</u> dose, every four hours. If symptoms are overwhelming, every TWO hours.

The Word works! WORK the Word!
Results guaranteed.

Psalm 103:20 (NKJV)

[20] Bless the LORD, you His angels, Who excel in strength, who do His word, Heeding the voice of His word.

Proverbs 4:20-22 (NKJV)

[20] My son, give attention to my words; Incline your ear to my sayings.

[21] Do not let them depart from your eyes; Keep them in the midst of your heart;

[22] For they *are* life to those who find them And health to all their flesh.

2 Corinthians 1:20 (NKJV)

[20] For all the promises of God in Him *are* Yes, and in Him Amen, to the glory of God through us.

Remember, if the enemy begins to tell you that it's not working, that's your key to hold fast to your confession of faith <u>without wavering</u>. You WILL possess the manifestation of your healing! Press toward the victory. It already belongs to you. Hallelujah!

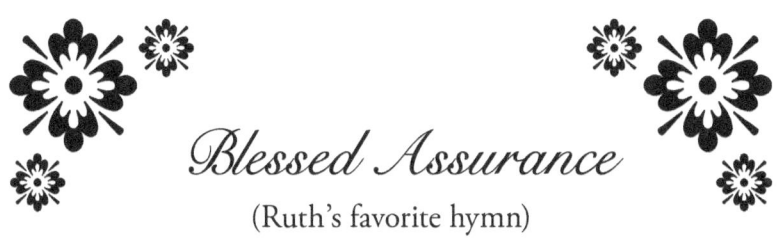

Blessed Assurance

(Ruth's favorite hymn)

1. Blessed assurance, Jesus is mine!
2. Oh, what a foretaste of glory divine!
3. Heir of salvation, purchase of God,
4. Born of His Spirit, washed in His blood.

> Refrain:
> This is my story, this is my song,
> Praising my Savior all the day long;
> This is my story, this is my song,
> Praising my Savior all the day long.

5. Perfect submission, perfect delight,
6. Visions of rapture now burst on my sight;
7. Angels, descending, bring from above
8. Echoes of mercy, whispers of love.

9. Perfect submission, all is at rest,
10. I in my Savior am happy and blest,
11. Watching and waiting, looking above,
12. Filled with His goodness, lost in His love.

Copyright: Public Domain

The lyrics were written in 1873 by Frances J. Crosby (1820 1915). The music was composed by her friend Phoebe P. Knapp (1839-1908).

The words were inspired by a bible verse.
[22]Let us draw near with a true heart in full assurance of faith, having our hearts sprinkled from an evil conscience, and our bodies washed with pure water. (Hebrews 10:22 KJV)

Postscript

As I put together this manuscript, recurring thoughts of our life together and of Ruth's battle with cancer kept going through my mind. Ruth and I were very active in our inner city church. Ruth sang in the praise and worship band and helped with vacation bible school. I ran the sound system for the praise team on Sundays and for special events. Our daughter participated in the dance troupe.

One particular Sunday service stands out in my mind. It was to be Ruth's last service although few knew that at the time. She was not able to stand for long periods and sang while seated during this service. Afterwards she was helped off the stage and was never strong enough to attend another service. But what I remember most about that last service was one of the songs which contained the lyrics, "He gives and takes away." I did not want to hear those words; that thought was just too hard to bear.

As Ruth grew weaker, I questioned why God would let this happen to Ruth. God, can't you spare Ruth from this cancer—from this pain and suffering? Of course the answer is YES but sometimes God has a different plan for us. He can use some of the hardest and most stressful times in our lives to draw us and those around us closer to Him.

Our church, Ruth's prayer groups, our family, myself and so many others prayed for Ruth's healing while she still walked on this earth. But God chose to take Ruth home with Him for her healing. God can and will take the sting out of death and the stress from life's burdens if we can just open our heart to His comforting spirit.

Whosoever believeth in Him shall not perish but will have eternal life. My family, friends and I miss Ruth as many others miss their loved ones. But please remember God has a plan for you as He did for me. He will give you the tools you need if only you ask—doors will be opened.

Ruth's faith in God never wavered. She prayed for healing here on earth but God chose to heal her in His arms.

As Ruth said, "Jesus shielded me with His love and kindness. He comforted me in the beginning and walked with me till the end. I am now resting in His arms."

I hope *This Is My Story* can help you in your walk with the Lord. Ruth's story has lifted me during many long days and nights. I miss Ruth and will always love her.

Steve

Blank Pages for Notes